The Flu Virus, Its Prevention and Vaccination Saga

Protecting Lives, Stopping Outbreaks, and the Future of Global Health Safety

Martin Cowel

Table of Contents

Introduction

Influenza, sometimes referred to as the flu, is a respiratory disease that is spread by influenza viruses. It can occasionally result in death as well as moderate to severe disease. Each year, the seasonal flu claims millions of lives globally and is a serious public health risk. Reducing the prevalence of this potentially fatal illness requires effective flu prevention and immunization.

The flu virus is extremely contagious and can be easily passed from person to person by droplets that are released when infected persons talk, sneeze, or cough. Additionally, it can be transferred by touching one's lips, nose, or eyes after coming into contact with surfaces or things that have the flu virus on them. Fever, chills, headache, sore throat, runny or stuffy nose, body aches, and exhaustion are some of the symptoms of the flu. The flu can occasionally result in consequences such sinus infections, pneumonia, bronchitis, and worsened existing medical issues.

Combining vaccination, public health initiatives, and good personal cleanliness are the three main ways to prevent the flu. Avoiding direct contact with sick people, covering up coughs and sneezes, and washing your hands frequently are all important preventative measures against the flu. Flu activity monitoring, early diagnosis and treatment, and flu vaccination promotion are examples of public health interventions.

The best defense against the flu and its effects is vaccination. Flu shots are intended to guard against the most prevalent types of the virus that are predicted to resurface every flu season. Every year, the flu vaccine's composition is examined and adjusted as necessary to reflect the viruses that are currently in circulation. Vaccines against the flu induce the production of antibodies by the immune system that guard against the virus. The body needs around two weeks following immunization in order to produce antibodies and offer protection.

The advantages of influenza vaccination go beyond the person who gets the shot. Herd immunity is created when a sizable section of the populace receives vaccinations; this stops the virus from spreading broadly and shields the most vulnerable people, including young children, the elderly, and those with compromised immune systems. Vaccination also lessens the strain on healthcare systems by lowering the number of hospital stays and doctor visits associated with the flu.

Flu vaccination rates are still below ideal in many populations, even though the vaccine is readily available and has been shown to be effective. Misconceptions about the flu and the vaccine, anxiety about side effects, lack of access to healthcare facilities, and a low perceived risk of getting the flu are common obstacles to getting vaccinated against it. Addressing these obstacles and raising immunization rates requires public health campaigns and educational initiatives.

Concerns regarding the possibility of the introduction of new, more deadly influenza viruses have increased in light of the recent advent of avian influenza (bird flu) strains like H5N1. Farmworkers are more likely to come into contact with avian influenza viruses due to their close proximity to poultry and other livestock. In an effort to lower the danger of farmworkers contracting bird flu and stop the creation of novel influenza strains through genetic reassortment, the US Centers for Disease Control and Prevention (CDC) has started to vaccinate farmworkers against the seasonal flu.

A key element of public health initiatives to lessen the effects of seasonal flu and avert possible pandemics is vaccination and flu prevention. We can shield people from the devastation caused by influenza by recognizing the significance of immunization, removing obstacles to vaccination, and putting specific public health programs into place.

Chapter 1: Understanding Influenza

Influenza, which is often known as the flu, is a virus-induced infectious disease. These viruses cause symptoms that can range from moderate to severe and, in rare circumstances, could be fatal. They infect the respiratory tract, which includes the nose, throat, and occasionally the lungs. For the purpose of creating efficient preventative and treatment plans, it is vital to comprehend the nature of the flu virus.

As members of the Orthomyxoviridae family, influenza viruses are distinguished by their distinct genetic makeup and structure. The virus has an encapsulated spherical diameter ranging from 80 to 120 nanometers. Its eight-segmented RNA genome, which permits substantial genetic reassortment and mutation, adds to the virus's capacity to elude the immune system.

The surface of the influenza virus is covered with two types of glycoproteins: hemagglutinin (HA) and neuraminidase (NA). These proteins are critical for the virus's ability to infect host cells and spread within the host. Hemagglutinin binds to receptors on the surface of respiratory epithelial cells, facilitating viral entry. Neuraminidase helps release new viral particles from infected cells, allowing the virus to spread to other cells and hosts.

The flu virus is highly contagious and spreads primarily through respiratory droplets when an infected person coughs, sneezes, or talks. It can also be transmitted by touching surfaces contaminated with the virus and then touching the face. The incubation period for the flu is typically one to four days, and infected individuals can spread the virus before they even show symptoms.

Symptoms of the flu include fever, chills, muscle aches, cough, congestion, runny nose, headaches, and fatigue. While most people recover within a few weeks, the flu can lead to severe complications, particularly in vulnerable populations such as young children, the elderly, and those with underlying health conditions. Complications can include pneumonia, bronchitis, sinus infections, and exacerbation of chronic diseases like asthma and heart disease.

Influenza has been responsible for numerous outbreaks and pandemics throughout history, with varying degrees of severity and impact on human populations. Understanding the history of influenza outbreaks provides valuable insights into the virus's behavior and the importance of public health interventions.

One of the earliest recorded influenza pandemics occurred in 1580, originating in Asia and spreading to Europe, Africa, and the Americas. Historical records describe a disease characterized by high fever and severe respiratory symptoms, with significant mortality rates. This pandemic highlighted the global reach and devastating potential of influenza.

The most notorious influenza pandemic in modern history is the Spanish flu of 1918-1919. It is estimated that the Spanish flu infected one-third of the world's population and caused the deaths of approximately 50 million people. The pandemic's high mortality rate was due in part to the virulence of the H1N1 influenza virus strain and the lack of effective medical interventions at the time. The Spanish flu disproportionately affected young adults, unlike typical seasonal flu, which primarily impacts the very young and the elderly.

The H2N2 virus that produced the 1957–1958 Asian flu and the H3N2 virus that caused the 1968–1969 Hong Kong flu are examples of subsequent influenza pandemics. Despite being less severe than the Spanish flu, both outbreaks caused a considerable amount of sickness and mortality on a global scale. Since then, the development of vaccinations and antiviral drugs has enhanced our capacity to control and lessen the effects of influenza pandemics.

The 2009 H1N1 pandemic, also known as the swine flu, was a stark reminder of the ongoing threat posed by influenza viruses. The H1N1 virus emerged from genetic reassortment involving influenza viruses from pigs, birds, and humans. It spread rapidly worldwide, leading to millions of infections and thousands of deaths. The global response to the H1N1 pandemic underscored the importance of surveillance, vaccination, and public health preparedness.

Types of Influenza Viruses

Influenza viruses are categorized into four types: A, B, C, and D. Each type has distinct characteristics and impacts human and animal health differently.

- Influenza A viruses are the most variable and are responsible for the most severe influenza pandemics and epidemics. These viruses infect humans, birds, pigs, horses, and other animals. Influenza A viruses are further subtyped based on the combination of hemagglutinin (HA) and neuraminidase (NA) proteins on their surface. For example, H1N1 and H3N2 are subtypes of influenza A that commonly circulate in humans. Influenza A viruses are known for their ability to undergo antigenic drift and shift, leading to significant genetic changes that can result in new strains and potentially cause pandemics.

2. Influenza B Viruses

- Influenza B viruses primarily infect humans and are less variable than influenza A viruses. They are not divided into subtypes but are categorized into two lineages:

B/Yamagata and B/Victoria. Influenza B viruses are responsible for seasonal flu epidemics and can cause significant illness, particularly in children and the elderly. However, they are generally less likely to cause pandemics compared to influenza A viruses.

3. Influenza C Viruses

- Influenza C viruses infect humans and pigs and typically cause mild respiratory illness. These viruses are less common and less well-studied than influenza A and B viruses. Influenza C infections are generally not associated with large outbreaks or severe disease.

4. Influenza D Viruses

- Influenza D viruses primarily infect cattle and are not known to infect humans. These viruses were identified more recently and are the least understood among the influenza virus types. While influenza D viruses do not pose a direct threat to human health, they are of interest in veterinary medicine and animal health.

For the development of successful vaccinations, therapies, and public health initiatives, an understanding of the many influenza virus strains and their behavior is essential. To detect novel strains of influenza viruses, track their progress, and address new dangers, ongoing research and surveillance are crucial.

Because influenza can result in severe complications, pandemics on occasion, and widespread disease, it continues to pose a serious threat to public health. The genetic heterogeneity and propensity for reassortment of the flu virus highlight its nature and emphasize the need for further research, surveillance, and vaccination campaigns. We can more effectively prepare for and lessen the effects of upcoming influenza epidemics and pandemics by studying the history of influenza outbreaks and comprehending the many influenza virus types.

Chapter 2: The Bird Flu Threat

A class of influenza viruses known as "bird flu," or "avian influenza," primarily affects birds but can also sporadically infect humans and other animals. The H5N1 virus is one of the most well-known and worrisome viruses. The influenza A virus subtype H5N1 is extremely pathogenic, which means it can result in serious illness and significant death rates, especially in birds.

The H5N1 virus first gained significant attention in the late 1990s when outbreaks were reported in poultry farms in Asia. The virus is particularly adept at infecting domestic birds such as chickens and ducks, leading to severe outbreaks that can devastate poultry populations. The virus spreads through direct contact with infected birds or contaminated surfaces, including water, feed, and equipment.

The structure of the H5N1 virus includes surface proteins hemagglutinin (H) and neuraminidase (N), which are crucial for the virus's ability to infect host cells and replicate. Hemagglutinin allows the virus to bind to receptors on the surface of host cells, facilitating entry, while neuraminidase helps release new viral particles from infected cells, enabling the virus to spread.

The impact of H5N1 on livestock is profound. Infected birds often exhibit severe symptoms such as respiratory distress, swelling, and a sudden drop in egg production. Mortality rates in affected flocks can be extraordinarily high, sometimes approaching 100%. This not only causes significant economic losses for farmers but also disrupts food supply chains, leading to broader economic and social consequences.

The economic impact of bird flu outbreaks can be staggering. In addition to the direct losses from the death of poultry, farmers and governments often have to implement culling programs to prevent the spread of the virus, further exacerbating economic losses. Trade restrictions and decreased consumer confidence can also affect the poultry industry, leading to financial strain on businesses and communities that rely on poultry farming.

Human infections with H5N1, while relatively rare, can be severe and often fatal. The first known human cases were reported in Hong Kong in 1997, where 18 people were infected, and six died. The primary mode of transmission to humans is through direct or close contact with infected birds or contaminated environments. Symptoms in humans can range from typical flu-like symptoms, such as fever and cough, to severe respiratory illness, pneumonia, and multi-organ failure.

The high mortality rate in human cases, which has been estimated at around 60%, is particularly concerning. The virus's ability to cause severe disease in humans and its potential to mutate and become more easily transmissible between humans raises fears of a possible pandemic. If H5N1 were to acquire the ability to spread efficiently from person to person, the consequences could be catastrophic, given the virus's lethality and the global population's lack of immunity.

Several notable outbreaks of H5N1 have occurred since it was first identified, each highlighting the virus's potential to cause widespread harm. One of the earliest significant outbreaks occurred in Hong Kong in 1997, when the virus infected poultry and humans. The swift response by Hong Kong authorities, which included the culling of all poultry in the territory, helped prevent a more extensive outbreak.

In 2003, H5N1 re-emerged in South Korea and subsequently spread to other Asian countries, including Vietnam, Thailand, and Indonesia. These outbreaks led to the deaths of millions of birds and numerous human fatalities. The virus continued to spread to parts of Europe, the Middle East, and Africa in subsequent years, demonstrating its ability to move across continents and affect diverse populations of birds and humans.

The 2004-2006 outbreak in Southeast Asia was particularly severe, with Vietnam, Thailand, and Indonesia experiencing significant human and poultry cases. The widespread nature of these outbreaks led to heightened surveillance and response measures globally, as countries recognized the need to contain the virus and prevent a potential pandemic.

In 2013, a new strain of H5N1 emerged in China, leading to human infections and fatalities. This strain was highly pathogenic in birds and had the potential to cause severe disease in humans. The outbreak prompted a renewed focus on surveillance and the development of vaccines and antiviral treatments to mitigate the threat of H5N1.

In addition to these major outbreaks, H5N1 has caused sporadic infections in birds and humans in various parts of the world. These incidents underscore the ongoing threat posed by the virus and the need for continued vigilance. The World Health Organization (WHO) and other international health agencies have emphasized the importance of monitoring and controlling H5N1 and other avian influenza viruses to prevent future outbreaks.

Efforts to combat H5N1 include vaccination programs for poultry, biosecurity measures to prevent the spread of the virus, and research into vaccines and treatments for human infections. Public health campaigns aim to raise awareness about the risks of avian influenza and promote practices that reduce the likelihood of transmission from birds to humans.

Despite these efforts, challenges remain. The virus's ability to mutate and adapt means that new strains can emerge, potentially with different characteristics and levels of virulence. The interconnected nature of global trade and travel also increases the risk of the virus spreading across borders, making it a global concern that requires coordinated international action.

The H5N1 form of avian flu, in particular, continues to pose a serious risk to human health and animals. Its capacity to infect humans and cause serious illness, along with its capacity to cause severe disease and high mortality rates in birds, highlight the significance of continued surveillance, research, and public health measures. Previous outbreaks have demonstrated the virus's potential to cause extensive harm and the necessity of taking strong precautions to stop and contain its spread. The threat posed by bird flu serves as a constant reminder of the need for readiness and alertness in the face of newly developing infectious illnesses, as global health concerns continue to change.

Chapter 3: The Role of Farmworkers

In the agricultural industry, farmworkers are vital to the production and availability of food. But they are frequently more vulnerable to a range of illnesses, including viral diseases like seasonal influenza and avian flu (H5N1). Their living arrangements and the type of employment they do greatly increase their susceptibility.

First of all, farmworkers usually come into touch with livestock, particularly poultry, which serves as a major bird flu viral reservoir. They come into contact with more infections when handling birds, maintaining animal waste, and cleaning coops. Via direct contact with diseased birds, their droppings, or contaminated surfaces, bird flu viruses can spread. The lack of proper protective gear among farmworkers increases their risk of infection.

Secondly, many farmworkers live in crowded and substandard housing conditions. These living environments can facilitate the spread of infectious diseases. Limited access to clean water, sanitation facilities, and proper hygiene practices exacerbates the risk of disease transmission. Additionally, the communal nature of their living conditions means that once an infection is introduced, it can spread rapidly among the residents.

Another factor contributing to the vulnerability of farmworkers is their often limited access to healthcare. Many farmworkers are immigrants or belong to marginalized communities, which can limit their access to medical services. Language barriers, lack of health insurance, and fear of immigration enforcement can prevent farmworkers from seeking medical care or receiving vaccinations. This lack of healthcare access makes it difficult for them to receive timely diagnoses and treatment, increasing the likelihood of severe outcomes from infections.

The daily challenges faced by farmworkers extend beyond their heightened risk of infectious diseases. The physical nature of their work exposes them to a range of occupational hazards. Farmwork often involves long hours of strenuous labor, frequently in harsh conditions. Exposure to extreme weather, such as intense heat or cold, can lead to heat-related illnesses, hypothermia, and other weather-related health issues.

Farmworkers are also at risk for injuries related to the use of heavy machinery and equipment. Accidents involving tractors, harvesters, and other machinery can result in serious injuries or fatalities. The repetitive nature of many farm tasks can lead to musculoskeletal disorders, such as back pain, joint problems, and repetitive strain injuries. These physical ailments can have long-term impacts on the health and well-being of farmworkers.

Pesticide exposure is another significant health risk for farmworkers. The use of pesticides in agriculture is common, and farmworkers often handle or are in close proximity to these chemicals. Pesticide exposure can lead to acute symptoms such as skin rashes, eye irritation, respiratory problems, and nausea. Long-term exposure has been linked to chronic health conditions, including cancer, reproductive issues, and neurological disorders. Unfortunately, many farmworkers are not provided with adequate protective equipment or training on safe pesticide use.

The mental health of farmworkers is also a critical concern. The stress and anxiety associated with job insecurity, financial instability, and immigration status can take a toll on their mental well-being. The isolation of working in remote rural areas and being separated from family and community support systems can exacerbate feelings of loneliness and depression. Mental health services are often lacking in rural areas, leaving farmworkers without the support they need to address these issues.

Given the myriad health risks faced by farmworkers, there is a pressing need for targeted health interventions to protect this vulnerable population. One of the primary areas of focus should be improving access to healthcare. Mobile health clinics and community health programs can bring medical services directly to farmworkers, bypassing some of the barriers they face in accessing traditional healthcare facilities. These programs can provide routine check-ups, vaccinations, and treatment for acute and chronic conditions.

Language and cultural barriers must also be addressed to ensure effective healthcare delivery. Healthcare providers should be trained in cultural competency and employ bilingual staff to communicate effectively with farmworkers. Outreach and education programs can help raise awareness about the importance of preventive care, such as vaccinations, and how to access available health services.

Workplace safety is another critical area for intervention. Employers should be required to provide adequate protective gear and training on safe work practices. This includes proper handling of machinery, safe use of pesticides, and measures to prevent heat-related illnesses. Regular safety inspections and enforcement of labor laws can help ensure that farmworkers are working in safe conditions.

Addressing housing conditions is also essential. Efforts should be made to improve the living conditions of farmworkers by providing access to clean water, sanitation facilities, and safe housing. Programs that offer affordable and safe housing options for farmworkers can significantly reduce their risk of infectious diseases and improve their overall quality of life.

Mental health support is another crucial aspect of health interventions for farmworkers.

Community-based mental health programs can provide counseling and support services to help farmworkers cope with the stresses and challenges of their work and personal lives. These programs should be accessible, confidential, and culturally sensitive to effectively meet the needs of farmworkers.

Vaccination programs are particularly important in the context of infectious diseases such as influenza. Targeted vaccination campaigns can help protect farmworkers from seasonal flu and reduce the risk of co-infection with bird flu viruses. Mobile vaccination units and vaccination drives at work sites and community centers can increase vaccine uptake among farmworkers. Educating farmworkers about the benefits of vaccination and addressing any misconceptions or fears they may have is also crucial for the success of these programs.

In addition to healthcare and safety measures, broader policy changes are needed to protect the health and rights of farmworkers. This includes advocating for labor rights, fair wages, and access to health insurance. Legal protections for immigrant farmworkers can help alleviate the fear of seeking medical care and ensure that they receive the support they need.

Despite being essential to the agricultural industry, farmworkers' living and working conditions pose serious health concerns. Targeted health interventions are necessary because of their increased risk of infectious diseases, work-related dangers, and restricted access to healthcare. Protecting the health and well-being of farmworkers requires a number of important actions, including expanding access to healthcare, guaranteeing job safety, resolving housing issues, offering mental health support, and putting immunization programs into place. In order to create a safer and healthier environment for this vulnerable population, broader legislative measures are also necessary to strengthen labor rights and give farmworkers legal safeguards.

Chapter 4: Vaccination as a Preventive Measure

One of the best methods for preventing infectious diseases, such as influenza, is vaccination. By lowering the frequency and severity of the flu, the flu vaccine helps to protect both individuals and communities. To fully appreciate the usefulness of seasonal flu vaccines in public health, one must have a thorough understanding of their development process, effectiveness, and safety.

Flu vaccines work by stimulating the immune system to recognize and fight the influenza virus. The vaccine introduces antigens, which are substances that trigger an immune response, to the body. These antigens are typically inactivated (killed) or weakened forms of the virus, or they might be proteins from the virus's surface. When the immune system encounters these antigens, it produces antibodies. These antibodies remain in the body and are ready to combat the actual virus if the person is exposed to it in the future.

The primary goal of the flu vaccine is to prompt the immune system to develop a memory of the virus without causing the disease itself. This process, known as immunization, helps ensure that the immune system can respond quickly and effectively to prevent illness or reduce its severity. Flu vaccines are designed to protect against the influenza strains predicted to be most prevalent in the upcoming flu season, based on global surveillance and research.

The development of seasonal flu vaccines is a complex and annual process that involves international collaboration among scientists, health organizations, and pharmaceutical companies. It begins with global surveillance of influenza activity. Researchers collect and analyze data on circulating flu strains from around the world. This information is used to predict which strains are likely to be most common during the next flu season.

Twice a year, the World Health Organization (WHO) convenes a meeting of experts to review the surveillance data and recommend which strains should be included in the flu vaccine for the upcoming season. These recommendations are based on factors such as the prevalence of specific strains, their geographic spread, and their potential to cause severe illness.

The process of making the vaccine starts as soon as the strains are chosen. Usually, this procedure begins six months in advance of flu season. There are various varieties of influenza vaccinations, such as:

- Inactivated Influenza Vaccines (IIVs): These vaccines contain killed viruses and are the most common type. They are usually administered via injection.
- Live Attenuated Influenza Vaccines (LAIVs): These vaccines contain weakened live viruses

and are typically given as a nasal spray. They are suitable for certain age groups and health conditions.

- Recombinant Influenza Vaccines (RIVs): These vaccines use recombinant DNA technology to produce viral proteins that stimulate an immune response. They are an alternative for individuals with egg allergies since they do not require egg-based production methods.

Purifying the viral components, creating the vaccine, and cultivating the chosen virus strains in eggs or cell cultures are the steps involved in manufacturing flu vaccines. Thorough quality control and testing guarantee the vaccines' safety and effectiveness prior to their distribution to healthcare practitioners.

The effectiveness of flu vaccines can vary from year to year, depending on several factors. One of the primary factors is the match between the vaccine strains and the circulating strains of the virus. If the vaccine strains closely match the prevalent strains, the vaccine's effectiveness tends to be higher. However, even when there is a less-than-perfect match, the vaccine can still provide significant protection by reducing the severity of illness and preventing complications.

Effectiveness also varies among different populations. Flu vaccines tend to be more effective in younger, healthy individuals and less effective in older adults and those with weakened immune systems. However, even in these populations, the vaccine can reduce the risk of severe outcomes such as hospitalization and death.

The safety of flu vaccines is rigorously monitored. Extensive clinical trials are conducted to evaluate the safety and efficacy of vaccines before they are approved for public use. These trials involve thousands of participants and are designed to identify any potential side effects. Once a vaccine is licensed, ongoing surveillance systems continue to monitor its safety in the general population.

Common side effects of flu vaccines are generally mild and temporary. They may include soreness at the injection site, low-grade fever, and muscle aches. Severe side effects are extremely rare. The benefits of vaccination, including reduced risk of flu-related complications and transmission, far outweigh the risks.

Public health agencies, such as the Centers for Disease Control and Prevention (CDC) and the WHO, strongly recommend annual flu vaccination for most people aged six months and older. Vaccination is especially important for high-risk groups, including young children, older adults, pregnant women, and individuals with chronic health conditions.

The mainstay of flu prevention and management is vaccination. In order to lower the risk of sickness and its complications, flu vaccinations function by preparing the immune system to identify and combat the virus. Choosing the most appropriate strains for each flu season is the goal of the careful and cooperative procedure that goes into developing seasonal flu vaccinations. Although there are differences in the efficacy of flu shots, their safety has been proved, and they are an essential component of maintaining public health. Reducing the impact of influenza on people and communities requires ensuring universal access to flu vaccinations and promoting vaccine uptake.

Chapter 5: The CDC's Initiative

The US Centers for Disease Control and Prevention (CDC) initiated a $5 million project to provide seasonal flu vaccines to livestock workers in response to growing worries about the possibility of coinfection between avian influenza (H5N1) and seasonal influenza among farmworkers. In an effort to reduce the hazards associated with the convergence of these two viruses—which may give rise to a new, more severe strain of influenza—this program is a proactive approach to public health.

The CDC's initiative is not merely a vaccination campaign; it is a comprehensive public health strategy that integrates vaccine distribution with education, outreach, and support services tailored to the needs of farmworkers. By focusing on a population at high risk of exposure to both human and avian influenza viruses, the CDC aims to prevent the emergence of a supercharged flu virus that could pose a significant threat to both human and animal health.

Goals and Objectives

The primary goal of the CDC's $5 million initiative is to protect the health and safety of farmworkers who are at increased risk of influenza virus coinfection due to their proximity to livestock and poultry. By vaccinating these workers against seasonal flu, the initiative aims to reduce the likelihood of genetic reassortment—a process where multiple influenza viruses infect a single host and exchange genetic material, potentially creating a new, more virulent strain.

Several specific objectives underpin this overarching goal:

- Reduce Influenza Incidence: By increasing vaccination rates among farmworkers, the initiative aims to lower the incidence of seasonal flu in this population, thereby reducing the overall burden of disease.

- Prevent Virus Coinfection: Vaccinating farmworkers against seasonal flu decreases the chances of coinfection with H5N1, reducing the risk of genetic reassortment and the emergence of a novel influenza virus.

- Enhance Public Health Preparedness: The initiative seeks to strengthen public health infrastructure by improving surveillance, vaccination delivery systems, and emergency response capabilities in areas with significant livestock farming activities.

- Promote Health Equity: Recognizing that farmworkers often face barriers to healthcare access, the initiative aims to ensure equitable access to vaccines and health services, addressing disparities that disproportionately affect this population.

- Increase Awareness and Education: Through targeted outreach and education efforts, the initiative aims to raise awareness about the importance of flu vaccination and promote understanding of the risks associated with influenza viruses.

Implementation Strategies

The CDC's initiative employs a multifaceted approach to achieve its goals, incorporating a range of strategies designed to maximize vaccine uptake and enhance public health outcomes. Key implementation strategies include:

- Community Engagement and Outreach: The initiative involves collaboration with community-based organizations, agricultural employers, and worker advocacy groups to reach farmworkers where they live and work. Mobile vaccination units, community events, and partnerships with local health departments are utilized to facilitate vaccine delivery and build trust within the community.

- Education and Training: To ensure farmworkers understand the importance of vaccination and the risks associated with influenza viruses, the initiative includes comprehensive education campaigns. These campaigns provide information on the benefits of flu vaccines, address common misconceptions, and offer guidance on how to access vaccination services. Training sessions for healthcare providers and outreach workers are also conducted to improve vaccine delivery and communication skills.

- Accessible Vaccination Services: The initiative prioritizes making vaccines accessible to farmworkers by offering them at convenient locations and times. Mobile clinics, pop-up vaccination sites at farms and agricultural centers, and collaborations with employers to provide on-site vaccinations are key components of this strategy. Additionally, efforts are made to reduce logistical barriers, such as transportation and language differences, to ensure that farmworkers can easily receive their vaccinations.

- Monitoring and Evaluation: To assess the effectiveness of the initiative and identify areas for improvement, the CDC implements robust monitoring and evaluation mechanisms. Data on vaccination rates, influenza incidence, and vaccine effectiveness are collected and analyzed. Feedback from farmworkers and community partners is also solicited to refine and enhance the program.
- Health Support Services: Recognizing that vaccination is just one aspect of health protection, the initiative includes additional support services for farmworkers. This includes access to testing, treatment, and personal protective equipment (PPE) for

those at risk of or exposed to H5N1. Providing comprehensive health services helps ensure that farmworkers receive the care they need to stay healthy and safe.

In the context of influenza prevention, the CDC's $5 million project is a proactive and planned response to the particular issues encountered by farmworkers. The effort constitutes a substantial investment in public health, since it tackles the dual objectives of preventing the formation of a novel influenza virus and fulfilling the urgent demand for seasonal flu vaccination. The efficacious execution of outreach, education, and vaccination tactics customized to the requirements of this susceptible demographic is important for its triumph.

The CDC's campaign serves as a reminder of how crucial focused public health actions are to preserving both individual and collective health. The program tries to lessen the possibility of a deadly new flu strain emerging by concentrating on farmworkers, a population that is more susceptible to influenza virus coinfection. The CDC strives to protect farmworkers' health and, by implication, the public's health through community involvement, education, easily available immunization services, and all-encompassing health assistance. This program emphasizes the vital role that proactive public health initiatives and preventative measures play in reducing the risks associated with infectious illnesses.

Chapter 6: The Science Behind Genetic Reassortment

Evolution of influenza viruses is largely dependent on the intricate process of genetic reassortment. One host cell becomes infected and exchanges genetic material when two or more distinct influenza virus strains do so. By combining genes from the original strains, this could lead to the development of a novel influenza virus. Because this method can result in the creation of new viruses with novel properties such as greater transmissibility, changed pathogenicity, or resistance to current antiviral medications and vaccines, it is especially important in the context of influenza viruses.

Influenza viruses are segmented RNA viruses, meaning their genomes are divided into distinct segments. This segmentation facilitates genetic reassortment, as segments from different viruses can be shuffled and recombined within a host cell. For instance, if a human cell is simultaneously infected by a human influenza virus and an avian influenza virus, the viral segments can mix, potentially producing a new virus with traits from both parent viruses.

The potential outcomes of genetic reassortment are varied. The new virus could be benign or it could pose significant public health challenges. The process of reassortment is largely random, but certain combinations of genes can give rise to viruses that are more adept at infecting humans, evading immune responses, or spreading rapidly. This unpredictability underscores the importance of monitoring and controlling influenza virus infections in both human and animal populations to mitigate the risks associated with reassortment.

Coinfection with multiple influenza viruses in a single host increases the risk of genetic reassortment. When a host is infected with more than one influenza strain, the probability of genetic material exchange and the emergence of a novel virus rises. This is particularly concerning in environments where humans are in close contact with animals, such as farms and live animal markets, where avian, swine, and human influenza viruses can coexist.

One significant risk of coinfection is the potential for the new virus to possess a combination of traits that make it particularly dangerous. For example, a reassortant virus could inherit the human-to-human transmissibility of a seasonal influenza virus and the virulence of an avian influenza virus like H5N1. Such a combination could lead to a highly transmissible and deadly influenza pandemic.

Moreover, the new virus might also acquire mutations that confer resistance to antiviral drugs or reduce the effectiveness of existing vaccines. This can complicate public health responses and necessitate the development of new vaccines and treatments. The dynamic nature of influenza viruses and their ability to rapidly evolve through genetic reassortment highlight the ongoing challenge of influenza prevention and control.

Another aspect of reassortment is its potential to create viruses with zoonotic potential, meaning they can jump from animals to humans. This zoonotic spillover is a key concern in influenza epidemiology, as it can introduce new influenza strains into the human population, leading to outbreaks or even pandemics. The 2009 H1N1 pandemic, for instance, was the result of a reassortment event involving influenza viruses from pigs, birds, and humans.

Historically, genetic reassortment has played a pivotal role in several major influenza pandemics.

One of the most notable examples is the 1957 H2N2 pandemic, also known as the Asian flu. This pandemic was caused by a reassortant virus that emerged from the combination of avian and human influenza viruses. The H2N2 virus had genes from both avian and human sources, enabling it to spread widely among humans with little preexisting immunity. The pandemic caused significant morbidity and mortality worldwide, highlighting the impact of reassortment on global health.

Another significant example is the 1968 H3N2 pandemic, also known as the Hong Kong flu. This pandemic virus resulted from reassortment between avian influenza viruses and the H2N2 human influenza virus. The H3N2 virus retained some genes from the H2N2 strain but acquired a new hemagglutinin (HA) gene from an avian virus, allowing it to evade human immune responses. The H3N2 virus continues to circulate as a seasonal influenza strain, demonstrating how reassortment can lead to long-term changes in the viral landscape.

The 2009 H1N1 pandemic, often referred to as the swine flu, provides a more recent example of genetic reassortment's implications. This virus emerged from a complex reassortment event involving influenza viruses from pigs, birds, and humans. The resultant H1N1 virus had segments from multiple sources, enabling it to infect humans and spread globally. The 2009 H1N1 pandemic underscored the importance of surveillance and preparedness, as it rapidly spread across the globe, affecting millions of people.

These historical examples illustrate the profound impact that genetic reassortment can have on influenza virus evolution and public health. Each pandemic caused by reassortant viruses has required substantial public health responses, including the development of new vaccines, antiviral treatments, and global surveillance efforts.

The lessons learned from these events continue to inform current influenza prevention and control strategies.

A crucial step in the evolution of influenza viruses is genetic reassortment, which has important consequences for public health. Comprehending the principles of reassortment, the potential hazards of coinfection, and the historical instances of reassortant viruses can contribute to the development of preventive and remedial measures for influenza outbreaks in the future. Addressing the persistent threat posed by influenza viruses and their capacity to quickly develop through genetic reassortment requires ongoing surveillance, immunization, and readiness.

Chapter 7: Public Health Strategies

In order to effectively address public health challenges, community-based approaches are essential, especially when working with communities who may face special risks or obstacles to receiving healthcare. For instance, farmworkers confront unique difficulties that call for specialized approaches to protect their health and safety. In order to conduct successful health interventions, these techniques emphasize building trust, utilizing local resources, and comprehending the needs of the community.

Community-based public health strategies involve working closely with local organizations, leaders, and members to develop and deliver health programs. This collaborative effort ensures that the interventions are culturally sensitive, accessible, and relevant to the community's specific circumstances. Engaging community stakeholders from the outset helps to build trust and ensures that the strategies are more likely to be accepted and sustained.

One effective community-based approach is the use of mobile health clinics. These clinics can travel to remote areas where farmworkers live and work, providing essential health services such as vaccinations, health screenings, and education. Mobile clinics overcome geographical barriers and make it easier for farmworkers to receive care without having to take time off work or travel long distances.

Another crucial aspect of community-based strategies is the involvement of community health workers (CHWs). CHWs are often members of the community they serve, which allows them to build rapport and trust with farmworkers. They can provide education, facilitate access to services, and support individuals in navigating the healthcare system. CHWs play a pivotal role in bridging the gap between farmworkers and healthcare providers.

Education is a cornerstone of effective public health strategies. For farmworkers, education programs must be designed to address their specific needs and circumstances. These programs should focus on raising awareness about health risks, preventive measures, and available health services, including vaccination programs.

Effective education programs use clear, simple language and culturally appropriate materials. This ensures that the information is easily understood and relevant. Visual aids, such as posters and pamphlets, can be particularly useful, as they can be displayed in workplaces and community centers where farmworkers gather.

In addition to providing information, education programs should engage farmworkers actively. Interactive workshops, discussions, and question-and-answer sessions can help to address any concerns or misconceptions. Involving farmworkers in the design and delivery of these programs can also increase their effectiveness. For example, farmworkers can share their experiences and insights, making the programs more relatable and impactful.

Peer education is another effective strategy. Farmworkers who receive training on health topics can educate their peers, creating a multiplier effect. Peer educators are often seen as more relatable and trustworthy, which can enhance the uptake of health messages.

Building trust is essential for the success of vaccination programs, particularly in communities that may have concerns or skepticism about vaccines. Trust is built through consistent, transparent communication and by demonstrating respect for the community's values and experiences.

One strategy to build trust is to involve respected community leaders and influencers in promoting vaccination. When these trusted figures endorse vaccines, it can have a powerful impact on community perceptions. For instance, farm owners, local religious leaders, or community organization heads can advocate for vaccination, helping to dispel myths and encourage uptake.

Addressing concerns and misinformation is also critical. Public health officials should provide clear, evidence-based information about the safety and effectiveness of vaccines. Open forums where farmworkers can ask questions and express their concerns can help to alleviate fears. It is important to acknowledge and address any past negative experiences with healthcare, as these can influence current attitudes toward vaccination.

Convenience and accessibility are key factors in building trust. Offering vaccinations at times and locations that are convenient for farmworkers demonstrates respect for their schedules and commitments. Mobile vaccination units, on-site clinics, and extended hours can make it easier for farmworkers to get vaccinated without disrupting their work.

Public health campaigns should also highlight the benefits of vaccination, not only for individual health but also for the community. Emphasizing how vaccines protect loved ones and contribute to the overall well-being of the community can be motivating factors for farmworkers to participate in vaccination programs.

Providing incentives can also be an effective strategy. Incentives could include items such as food vouchers, transportation assistance, or small financial rewards. These incentives not only make it easier for farmworkers to access vaccination services but also show appreciation for their participation.

Collaborating with employers is another important aspect of building trust. Employers can support vaccination efforts by providing paid time off for vaccinations, facilitating on-site vaccination clinics, and encouraging their workers to get vaccinated. When employers are actively involved in promoting and supporting vaccination, it reinforces the importance of the initiative.

Monitoring and evaluation are essential to ensure the effectiveness of these strategies. Regular feedback from farmworkers can help to identify any barriers or areas for improvement. Public health officials should be responsive to this feedback and willing to adapt their approaches as needed.

Community-based approaches to public health, especially in educating and engaging farmworkers and building trust in vaccination programs, are essential for effective health interventions. These strategies must be culturally sensitive, accessible, and tailored to the unique needs of the community.

Build trust and boost vaccination rates among farmworkers by incorporating community members, resolving concerns, offering pertinent and clear education, and guaranteeing convenience and accessibility.

Chapter 8: Case Studies and Real-World Applications

Public health initiatives implemented in the real world frequently result in success stories that can be useful models for similar programs in the future. The deployment of mobile health clinics in the Central Valley of California, which sought to offer farmworkers comprehensive healthcare services, including immunizations, is one noteworthy success story. By dramatically raising farmworkers' immunization rates, these clinics helped to lower the prevalence of the flu and other infections that may have been avoided.

The mobile clinics were equipped with medical staff who provided vaccinations, health screenings, and educational materials. By bringing healthcare services directly to the fields, these clinics overcame barriers such as transportation and time constraints that typically hinder farmworkers' access to healthcare. The program's success was largely due to its ability to meet farmworkers where they were, offering services at convenient times, including early mornings and late evenings.

Another success story is the community health worker (CHW) program in Texas. This program trained farmworkers to become health advocates within their communities. CHWs were instrumental in disseminating information about the importance of vaccinations, debunking myths, and guiding their peers to available health services. The personal connections and trust CHWs established with their communities led to higher vaccination uptake and overall better health outcomes.

While success stories are inspiring, they often come with challenges that offer critical lessons for future public health initiatives. One common challenge is overcoming vaccine hesitancy among farmworkers. Misinformation, cultural beliefs, and past negative experiences with healthcare can all contribute to reluctance to receive vaccinations. Addressing these concerns requires persistent efforts in education, transparent communication, and the involvement of trusted community figures.

The mobile health clinic program in California faced logistical challenges, such as securing funding, maintaining a consistent schedule, and ensuring the availability of medical supplies. Flexibility and adaptability were key in addressing these issues. For instance, the program had to adjust routes and schedules based on the agricultural calendar and weather conditions, demonstrating the importance of being responsive to the unique needs of the farmworker population.

In Texas, the CHW program initially struggled with retention and burnout among health workers. To mitigate this, the program introduced support mechanisms, including regular training sessions, mental health resources, and opportunities for professional development. These measures helped maintain a motivated and effective workforce, highlighting the need for robust support systems in community-based health programs.

Another lesson learned is the importance of data collection and analysis. Accurate data on vaccination rates, health outcomes, and program impact is crucial for evaluating effectiveness and securing ongoing funding. Both the California and Texas programs invested in robust data collection systems, which allowed them to demonstrate their success and make informed adjustments to their strategies.

Public health efforts to increase vaccination rates among farmworkers are ongoing and evolving. Building on the success of mobile clinics and CHW programs, new initiatives are exploring innovative ways to enhance healthcare delivery and engagement with farmworker communities.

One promising area is the integration of technology in public health efforts. Mobile health apps, for example, can provide farmworkers with up-to-date information on vaccination schedules, locations of mobile clinics, and health tips. These apps can also facilitate appointment scheduling and reminders, making it easier for farmworkers to stay on top of their health needs.

In addition to technology, partnerships with agricultural businesses are being strengthened. Employers play a crucial role in supporting the health of their workers. Collaborative programs that involve employers in health initiatives, such as on-site vaccination drives and health education workshops, are being expanded. These partnerships not only improve health outcomes but also enhance worker satisfaction and productivity.

Another focus area is the mental health and well-being of farmworkers. Recognizing that health is holistic, ongoing efforts are incorporating mental health services into existing programs. This includes providing access to counseling, stress management resources, and peer support groups. Addressing mental health alongside physical health ensures a more comprehensive approach to the well-being of farmworkers.

Looking to the future, public health officials are planning to scale successful models to other regions with large farmworker populations. Sharing best practices, resources, and training materials across states can help replicate the success seen in places like California and Texas. National and regional conferences, workshops, and collaborative networks are being developed to facilitate this knowledge exchange.

Moreover, policy reform lobbying will always be a crucial part of future initiatives. The goals of public health advocates are to guarantee improved working conditions, increase access to healthcare, and win more stable funding for farmworker health programs. The goal of legislative measures is to address the systemic obstacles that farmworkers encounter, such as lack of healthcare coverage and concerns with immigration status that affect access.

Insights into the achievements, difficulties, and lessons gained are provided via case studies and practical implementations of public health initiatives for farmworkers. A substantial beneficial impact can be achieved when activities are customized to the specific requirements of farmworker communities, as seen by the success stories of mobile health clinics and CHW programs. Nonetheless, obstacles including reluctance to receive vaccinations, logistical problems, and employee retention emphasize the necessity of adaptability, strong data collecting, and support systems. To maintain and broaden the impact of these essential public health programs, ongoing efforts are concentrated on integrating technology, bolstering employer relationships, treating mental health, and pushing for legislation changes. Public health officials may guarantee that farmworkers receive complete care and assistance by building on these experiences and consistently adapting to evolving requirements.

Chapter 9: Global Implications

A persistent worry in the field of global health is the possibility of a pandemic, especially with regard to influenza viruses. Pandemics caused by influenza arise from newly discovered virus strains that are highly contagious and can infect large numbers of people. The terrible effects that influenza pandemics may have on people, economies, and healthcare systems worldwide are shown by the history of pandemics, including the Asian flu of 1957, the Spanish flu of 1918, and the H1N1 pandemic of 2009.

Bird flu (H5N1) and other avian influenza viruses present a particularly concerning pandemic threat. These viruses primarily infect birds but can occasionally jump to humans, especially those who have close contact with infected poultry. While human-to-human transmission of H5N1 has been rare, the potential for the virus to mutate or reassort with human influenza viruses could lead to a highly transmissible and potentially deadly new strain. The theoretical risk of genetic reassortment—where multiple influenza viruses infect a single host and exchange genetic material—adds to the urgency of monitoring and controlling avian flu outbreaks.

The global interconnectedness of modern society means that an emerging influenza virus can spread rapidly across borders. International travel, trade, and human migration can facilitate the swift movement of pathogens, making early detection and response critical. A new pandemic strain could overwhelm healthcare systems, disrupt economies, and cause significant morbidity and mortality worldwide. Therefore, preparedness and proactive measures are essential to mitigate the impact of a potential influenza pandemic.

Effective response to the threat of a pandemic requires robust international cooperation. No single country can address the complex challenges posed by an emerging infectious disease alone. International organizations such as the World Health Organization (WHO) play a crucial role in coordinating global efforts to detect, prevent, and respond to influenza outbreaks.

The WHO's Global Influenza Surveillance and Response System (GISRS) is a network of laboratories and public health institutions that monitors influenza activity worldwide. This network enables the timely sharing of information about emerging strains, which is vital for tracking the spread of the virus and identifying potential pandemic threats. Collaborative research and data sharing through GISRS help in the development of vaccines and antiviral drugs tailored to combat specific influenza strains.

International cooperation also extends to joint exercises and simulations designed to test and improve pandemic preparedness plans. Countries participate in these exercises to evaluate their response capabilities, identify gaps, and enhance coordination among national and international stakeholders. These efforts ensure that, in the event of a pandemic, countries can act swiftly and effectively to contain the virus and minimize its impact.

Trade and travel restrictions, while often necessary during outbreaks, require careful coordination to avoid unnecessary economic disruption and ensure that essential goods and services continue to flow. International agreements and frameworks, such as the International Health Regulations (IHR), provide guidelines for managing public health risks while balancing the need for global mobility and commerce.

Preparing for future outbreaks involves a multi-faceted approach that includes surveillance, research, public health infrastructure, and community engagement. Surveillance systems must be capable of detecting new influenza strains quickly and accurately. This requires investment in laboratory capacity, training for health professionals, and the use of advanced technologies such as genomic sequencing to identify and track viral mutations.

Research is critical for developing vaccines, antiviral drugs, and other medical countermeasures. Continuous efforts are needed to improve the efficacy and production capacity of influenza vaccines. Universal flu vaccines, which aim to provide broad protection against multiple strains of the virus, are a promising area of research that could significantly enhance pandemic preparedness.

Public health infrastructure must be robust and resilient to respond to outbreaks effectively. This includes ensuring adequate healthcare facilities, stockpiling essential supplies, and maintaining a trained and ready workforce. Public health campaigns should educate communities about preventive measures, such as vaccination and personal hygiene, and promote trust in health authorities.

Engaging communities is vital for effective outbreak response. Public trust in health authorities and adherence to public health recommendations can significantly influence the course of an outbreak. Transparent communication, culturally appropriate messaging, and involving community leaders in public health efforts can enhance compliance with preventive measures and vaccination programs.

Countries must also consider the social and economic impacts of pandemic preparedness. Policies should address the needs of vulnerable populations, ensure access to healthcare for all, and support economic recovery efforts in the aftermath of an outbreak. Social safety nets, economic stimulus packages, and support for small businesses are essential components of a comprehensive preparedness strategy.

Internationally, strengthening health systems in low- and middle-income countries is crucial. These countries often face greater challenges in outbreak response due to limited resources and infrastructure. International aid, capacity-building initiatives, and technology transfer can help bridge these gaps and enhance global pandemic preparedness.

Pandemic risk carries substantial worldwide ramifications, necessitating a well-coordinated and all-encompassing response. Effective preparedness requires strong public health infrastructure, research, surveillance, and international collaboration. The international community can lessen the effects of influenza pandemics and safeguard public health globally by taking lessons from previous outbreaks and investing in future capabilities. To make sure that the world is more ready for the next pandemic threat, governments, international organizations, and communities must work together.

Chapter 10: Moving Forward

Strengthening preventative measures continues to be a key component of public health policy as the world faces new and continuing health concerns. In order to slow the spread of infectious diseases and lessen their effects on people and communities, effective prevention is essential. This calls for a multifaceted strategy that includes bolstering health systems and developing novel vaccines.

Advancements in vaccine development are key to improving preventive measures and combating infectious diseases. Traditional vaccine development methods, which often involve growing viruses in laboratories and inactivating them, have been instrumental in creating effective vaccines. However, recent innovations are expanding the possibilities and accelerating the development process.

One major innovation is the use of mRNA technology. The success of mRNA vaccines in responding to the COVID-19 pandemic has demonstrated their potential. Unlike traditional vaccines, mRNA vaccines do not contain live virus but use a snippet of genetic material to instruct cells to produce a protein that triggers an immune response. This technology can be rapidly adapted to address new and emerging pathogens. For instance, researchers are exploring mRNA vaccines for influenza and other diseases, aiming to create more effective and versatile vaccines.

Another promising development is the concept of universal vaccines. Traditional flu vaccines must be updated annually to match circulating strains, which can be a slow and complex process. Universal vaccines aim to provide broad protection against multiple strains of a virus, reducing the need for annual updates and improving long-term protection. Research into universal influenza vaccines is progressing, with the goal of creating vaccines that offer year-round immunity against various influenza strains.

Nanotechnology is also playing a role in vaccine innovation. Nanoparticles can be used to create more stable and effective vaccines by enhancing the delivery and targeting of antigens. This technology can potentially improve vaccine efficacy and reduce the frequency of doses required, making vaccination programs more efficient and accessible.

Adjuvants, substances that enhance the body's immune response to a vaccine, are another area of innovation. New adjuvants can improve the effectiveness of vaccines by boosting the immune response, particularly in populations with weaker immune systems, such as the elderly. Research is focused on developing adjuvants that are both safe and effective, offering greater protection against infectious diseases.

Strengthening health systems is essential for effective disease prevention and response. A robust health system ensures that preventive measures, including vaccines, are accessible to all populations and that health services are capable of managing outbreaks and providing care.

One critical aspect of strengthening health systems is improving healthcare infrastructure. This includes building and maintaining healthcare facilities, equipping them with modern technologies, and ensuring that they are staffed with trained professionals. Investments in infrastructure help ensure that health services are available and efficient, particularly in underserved and remote areas.

Health systems must also focus on enhancing surveillance and data collection. Effective surveillance systems are crucial for early detection of outbreaks and monitoring disease trends. Investing in data collection technologies, such as electronic health records and real-time reporting systems, improves the ability to track and respond to health threats promptly.

Training and capacity-building for healthcare workers are vital components of strengthening health systems. Healthcare professionals must be equipped with the knowledge and skills needed to implement preventive measures, administer vaccines, and manage outbreaks. Ongoing training programs and professional development opportunities ensure that healthcare workers stay updated on the latest practices and technologies.

Equitable access to healthcare services is another critical area for improvement. Health systems must address disparities in access to preventive measures, such as vaccines, by ensuring that services are available to all individuals, regardless of their socioeconomic status. Community outreach programs, mobile health units, and partnerships with local organizations can help reach underserved populations and increase vaccination rates.

Public health education and community engagement are essential for promoting preventive measures and fostering trust in health systems. Educating the public about the importance of vaccination and other preventive practices helps encourage participation in vaccination programs and adherence to health recommendations. Engaging community leaders and utilizing culturally appropriate messaging can enhance the effectiveness of public health campaigns.

Looking ahead, the integration of technological advancements and innovative practices into health systems will be crucial for enhancing preventive measures. Digital health tools, such as telemedicine and health apps, can improve access to healthcare services and facilitate preventive care. By leveraging technology, health systems can provide more personalized and timely interventions, enhancing the overall effectiveness of preventive measures.

Collaboration between governments, international organizations, and the private sector will be essential for advancing vaccine development and strengthening health systems. Public-private partnerships can drive innovation, improve access to vaccines, and support global health initiatives. Collaborative efforts will also help address health disparities and ensure that preventive measures are accessible to all populations.

A comprehensive strategy for improving preventive measures is needed going ahead, including improvements in vaccine research and fortifying health systems. Novel approaches to fighting infectious diseases, like universal vaccinations and mRNA vaccines, are being presented by developments in vaccine technology. Enhancing health systems via fair access, training, surveillance, and infrastructure guarantees that preventative interventions are widely available and successfully applied. By concentrating on these areas, we may enhance public health outcomes and protect people globally by better anticipating and responding to health problems.

www.ingramcontent.com/pod-product-compliance
Lightning Source LLC
Chambersburg PA
CBHW081447250726
48662CB00009B/2984